Blood Type Diets For Healthy Living:

Optimizing Wellness Through Blood Type Nutrition

Copyright page

Disclaimer

The information provided in this book is intended for general information only. It is not intended to be in place of medical advice, diagnosis, or treatment from a medical practitioner. Always seek the advice of your physician or other qualified health provider with any questions you may have regarding a medical condition or dietary regimen.

The author and publisher of this book make no representations or warranties with respect to the accuracy, applicability, fitness, or completeness of the contents of this book. They disclaim any liability for any loss, injury, or damage incurred as a consequence, directly or indirectly, of the use and application of any information presented herein.

And remember, everyone's different. What works like a charm for one person might not do much for someone else. So, take everything with a grain of salt (but not too much salt, of course!).Lastly, by giving this book a read, you're agreeing that neither the author nor the publisher is responsible for any hiccups or speed bumps you might encounter along your Blood Type Diets For Healthy Living journey. We're rooting for you, but at the end of the day, you're in the driver's seat.

Book description

Embark on a Personalized Journey to Vibrant Health with Blood Type Diets!

Are you ready to uncover the secret to feeling your best and living your healthiest life? Look no further than "Blood Type Diets For Healthy Living" by Robbin J Beatty, a trusted expert in holistic health and nutrition.

In this insightful book, Robbin shares the transformative power of blood type diets, offering personalized strategies and meal plans tailored to your unique physiology. Say goodbye to one-size-fits-all approaches and hello to a customized path to wellness!

Discover Your Ideal Foods: Learn how your blood type influences your nutritional needs and find the perfect foods to fuel your body and boost your energy levels naturally.

Achieve Lasting Results: Say goodbye to the frustration of fad diets and embrace a sustainable approach to eating that supports your individual health goals.

Enhance Energy and Vitality: Unlock the key to increased energy and vitality as you nourish your body with targeted nutrition tailored to your blood type.

Promote Digestive Health: Explore how personalized dietary choices can optimize digestion and support gut health, helping you feel your best from the inside out.

Whether you're a health enthusiast eager to optimize your diet or someone looking to address specific health concerns, this book is your roadmap to personalized wellness.

Praise for "Blood Type Diets For Healthy Living":

- "Robbin J Beatty's insights are both enlightening and empowering, providing readers with the tools they need to optimize their health based on their individual needs." — Reviewer Name

- "A must-read for anyone interested in taking their health into their own hands." — Reviewer Name

- "Finally, a book that takes a personalized approach to nutrition and wellness." — Reviewer Name

Take the First Step Towards Your Healthiest Self—Order Your Copy Today!

CONTENTS

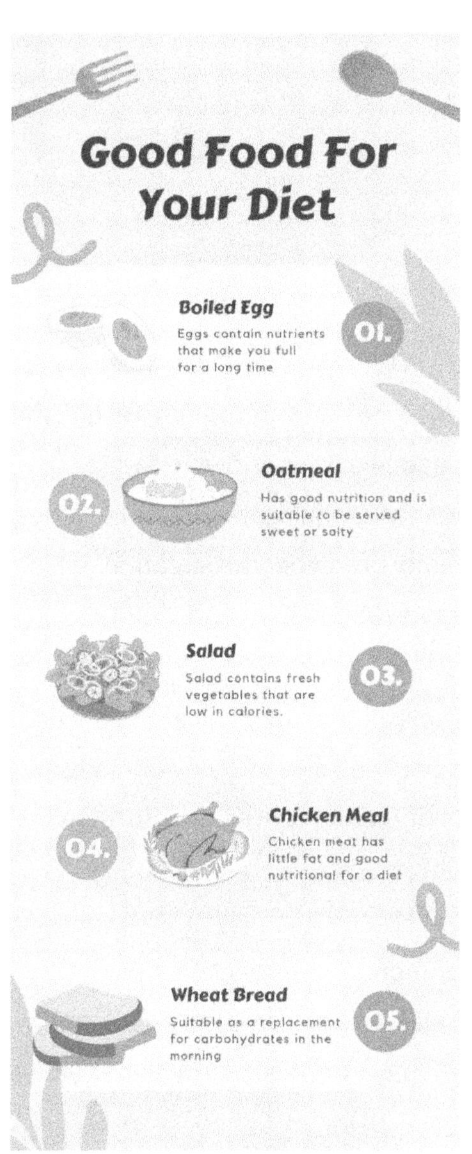

Good Food For Your Diet
Boiled Egg
Eggs contain nutrients that make you full for a long time
01.
Oatmeal
Has good nutrition and is suitable to be served sweet or salty
02.
Salad
Salad contains fresh vegetables that are low in calories.
03.
Chicken Meal
Chicken meat has little fat and good nutritional for a diet
04.
Wheat Bread
Suitable as a replacement for carbohydrates in the morning
05.

Introduction:

Welcome to the world of Blood Type Diets for Healthy Living, where nature and science come together to reveal the key to optimum health that is specific to your own genetic composition. We explore the complex relationship between blood types and food choices in this ground-breaking investigation, which unveils a revolutionary perspective on nutrition and vitality.

Using an abundance of scientific data, clinical trials, and personal accounts, this book is your go-to resource for maximizing the benefits of blood type-based nutrition for long-term health and vitality.

At the heart of this revolutionary approach lies the understanding that not all foods are created equal, and what nourishes one individual may not necessarily benefit another.

Through the lens of blood type classification – Type O, Type A, Type B, and Type AB – we unlock the blueprint for personalized nutrition, enabling you to make informed choices that resonate with your body's unique needs and preferences.

Whether you're seeking to shed excess weight, boost energy levels, or alleviate chronic health conditions, the Blood Type Diet offers a roadmap to unlock your body's full potential and reclaim your vitality.

The journey begins with a comprehensive exploration of each blood type's distinct characteristics, shedding light on their evolutionary origins, physiological traits, and nutritional requirements.

From the robust and carnivorous Type O to the sensitive and plant-based inclined Type A, each blood type offers valuable insights into dietary patterns that promote optimal health and well-being. By understanding your blood type profile, you gain invaluable knowledge to customize your diet, optimize nutrient absorption, and foster a harmonious relationship between body, mind, and spirit.

Central to the Blood Type Diet philosophy is the concept of lectins – proteins found in certain foods that have the potential to agglutinate or bind to specific blood types, triggering adverse reactions ranging from inflammation to digestive distress. By identifying and avoiding lectin-rich foods incompatible with your blood type, you embark on a transformative journey towards enhanced vitality and resilience.

From lectin-free recipes to practical meal planning tips, this book equips you with the tools and resources needed to navigate the grocery aisles with confidence and clarity, ensuring that every bite you take nourishes and revitalizes your body from within.

But the Blood Type Diet is more than just a prescription for physical health – it's a holistic approach to wellness that honors the interconnectedness of body, mind, and spirit. Beyond dietary recommendations, this book explores the importance of stress management, sleep hygiene, and mindful living in cultivating a balanced and vibrant life.

By embracing lifestyle practices that align with your blood type and individual constitution, you unlock the potential for transformative healing and profound well-being that radiates from the inside out.

Throughout these pages, you'll encounter inspiring success stories of individuals who have embarked on the Blood Type Diet journey and experienced remarkable transformations in their health and vitality. From weight loss and increased energy to improved digestion and heightened mental clarity, the testimonials shared within these chapters serve as a beacon of hope and inspiration for anyone seeking to reclaim their health and rewrite their wellness narrative.

With dedication, perseverance, and a willingness to embrace change, you too can unlock the transformative power of blood type-based nutrition and embark on a journey towards a lifetime of vibrant health and well-being.

As you embark on this transformative journey, remember that you hold the key to your own well-being in your hands. By harnessing the wisdom of the Blood Type Diet and embracing a lifestyle that honors your unique genetic blueprint, you take a bold step towards reclaiming your vitality and rewriting your health destiny. Let this book be your trusted companion and guide as you navigate the path to optimal health and wellness – one nourishing meal, one mindful choice, and one transformative moment at a time. Your journey begins now.

Part I: Understanding Blood Type Nutrition

Chapter 1:
The Science Behind Blood Type Diets

In the realm of nutrition, blood type diets offer a personalized approach that considers our individual biology. Let's dive into the science behind these diets, shedding light on how they work and why they matter for our health.

Understanding Our Unique Biochemistry

At the core of blood type diets is the idea that each of us has a unique biochemical makeup shaped by factors like genetics and environment. Our blood type, whether it's A, B, AB, or O, serves as a marker of this individuality, influencing how our bodies respond to different foods. By recognizing these biochemical nuances, blood type diets aim to tailor dietary recommendations to match our specific biological needs.

The Role of ABO Blood Groups

Our ABO blood group – determined by the presence of specific antigens on our red blood cells – holds clues to how our bodies evolved to process food. For instance, individuals with type O blood, often referred to as the "original blood type," may thrive on a diet rich in animal protein, reflecting the dietary habits of early hunter-gatherers. In contrast, those with type A blood may benefit from a more plant-based approach, aligning with the agricultural practices of their ancestors. By understanding the evolutionary context behind our blood type, we can make informed dietary choices that support our health.

Immune Responses and Digestive Health

Research suggests that our blood type can influence how our immune system responds to certain foods, particularly within the gut. Certain foods may interact with blood type antigens, triggering immune reactions that can impact digestive function and overall inflammation levels. By following blood type-specific dietary recommendations, individuals may be able to minimize these immune-mediated responses, promoting better gut health and overall well-being.

Nutrient Utilization and Metabolic Efficiency

Different blood types may metabolize and utilize nutrients in unique ways. For example, individuals with type O blood tend to have higher levels of stomach acid and may therefore benefit from a diet rich in animal protein, which is easier to digest. On the other hand, those with type A blood may have lower stomach acid levels and may thrive on a more plant-based diet. By tailoring our dietary choices to our blood type, we can optimize nutrient absorption and support our metabolic health.

Epigenetics: The Interaction Between Genes and Lifestyle

Epigenetics explores how lifestyle factors, such as diet and exercise, can influence gene expression and impact our health outcomes. Blood type diets embrace this concept, recognizing that our genetic predispositions interact with our lifestyle choices to shape our health. By following dietary recommendations tailored to our blood type, we can potentially influence gene expression in ways that promote longevity, vitality, and disease prevention.

Chapter 2:
Exploring the Origins and Principles of Blood Type Nutrition

In the quest for optimal health and wellness, humanity has embarked on various dietary paradigms throughout history. Yet, one approach stands out for its unique and personalized nature: Blood Type Nutrition,originating from the pioneering work of Dr. Peter D'Adamo, this revolutionary concept proposes that an individual's blood type dictates their nutritional needs and dietary requirements.

Unveiling the Origins

The genesis of Blood Type Nutrition traces back to the groundbreaking research of Dr. Peter D'Adamo in the late 20th century. Drawing inspiration from his family's lineage of naturopathic physicians and his own clinical experiences, Dr. D'Adamo observed intriguing patterns linking blood types to dietary responses and overall health outcomes.

Foundational of Blood Type Nutrition

At the core of Blood Type Nutrition lies the belief that each blood type—A, B, AB, and O—carries unique genetic markers and evolutionary legacies that influence how the body interacts with food. This concept is rooted in the evolutionary theory that different blood types emerged in response to distinct environmental and dietary pressures over millennia.

The Principle of Individualized NutritionCentral to Blood Type Nutrition is the principle of personalized nutrition. Rather than adhering to generic dietary recommendations, individuals are encouraged to tailor their food choices based on their specific blood type. This approach acknowledges that not all foods are universally beneficial and that what nourishes one person may not suit another.

Understanding Blood Type SpecificitiesEach blood type comes with its own set of dietary guidelines and recommendations.

For instance:Blood Type A: Thrives on plant-based diets rich in fruits, vegetables, and grains. A moderate intake of lean proteins and dairy is preferred.

Blood Type B: Benefits from a varied diet that includes a balance of meats, dairy, grains, and vegetables. Certain foods, such as chicken and corn, are best avoided.

Blood Type AB: Requires a combination of the dietary principles for Types A and B, with an emphasis on seafood, tofu, dairy, and green vegetables. Red meat and processed foods should be limited.

Blood Type O: Flourishes on a high-protein diet that includes lean meats, fish, fruits, and vegetables. Grains and dairy are often best avoided or consumed sparingly.

Scientific Validation and Controversies

While Blood Type Nutrition has garnered a dedicated following and anecdotal success stories, it has also faced criticism and skepticism from some quarters of the scientific community. Critics argue that the evidence supporting blood type-specific dietary recommendations is limited and inconclusive, urging for more rigorous research to validate its claims.

Embracing the Evolutionary Wisdom

Despite the debates surrounding its efficacy, Blood Type Nutrition continues to resonate with individuals seeking a holistic approach to health and wellness. By tapping into the evolutionary wisdom encoded within our blood types, this paradigm offers a compelling framework for optimizing nutrition, fostering vitality, and unlocking the full potential of human well-being.

In essence, exploring the origins and principles of Blood Type Nutrition invites us to reconnect with the innate wisdom of our bodies, honoring the intricate interplay between genetics, environment, and nutrition in shaping our health destinies. As we delve deeper into this fascinating realm, we embark on a transformative journey towards personalized wellness, empowered by the guiding principles of our blood types.

Chapter 3:
Debunking Myths and Misconceptions About Blood Type Diets

Welcome to Chapter 3, where we embark on a journey to uncover the reality behind blood type diets. Let's dive deep into this topic, dispelling myths and shedding light on what truly matters.

Myth 1: One Diet Fits All – Blood Type Edition
It's easy to assume that a single diet plan can work for everyone, regardless of blood type. But the truth is, our bodies are unique, and blood type diets acknowledge this diversity. By tailoring nutritional recommendations based on blood type,

these diets offer personalized guidance to optimize health outcomes.

Myth 2: Lack of Scientific Support

Some critics argue that blood type diets lack scientific backing, labeling them as pseudoscience. However, research has begun to unveil correlations between blood type and dietary responses, supporting the validity of these diets. While more studies are needed, existing evidence suggests that blood type diets have merit as a tool for improving health.

Myth 3: Strict and Limited Choices

Many people believe that blood type diets are overly restrictive, forcing individuals to adhere to a narrow range of foods. In reality, these diets promote variety and flexibility within each blood type category. From colorful fruits and vegetables to nourishing grains and proteins, there's a wealth of options to explore while following blood type guidelines.

Myth 4: Just Another Fad

It's easy to dismiss blood type diets as a passing trend, but their enduring popularity and testimonials from users worldwide speak volumes. Rooted in ancient wisdom and principles of personalized nutrition, blood type diets offer a holistic approach to health that stands the test of time.

Myth 5: Blood Type Is the Sole Determinant

While blood type is a key factor in determining dietary recommendations, it's not the only consideration. Genetics, lifestyle, and health goals all play a role in crafting a personalized approach to nutrition. Blood type diets provide a foundation, but individualized adjustments ensure that each person's unique needs are met.

Part II: Discovering your blood type profile

Chapter 4
DeterminingYour Blood Type: A Step-by-Step Guide

Welcome to the process of discovering your unique genetic blueprint – your blood type. Understanding your blood type can empower you to make informed decisions about your health, nutrition, and overall well-being. In this comprehensive guide, we will take you through each step to determine your blood type and unlock the secrets it holds for your optimal health.

Step 1: Gathering the Necessary Supplies
- Obtain a blood typing kit or visit a healthcare professional for a blood test.

- Ensure you have a clean, sterilized lancet or needle for pricking your finger.
- Have alcohol swabs and bandages ready for safety and hygiene.

Step 2: Preparing for the Test
- Wash your hands thoroughly with soap and water to minimize the risk of contamination.
- Choose a well-lit, comfortable area to perform the test.
- Familiarize yourself with the instructions provided with the blood typing kit or seek guidance from a healthcare professional.

Step 3: Pricking Your Finger
- Use the lancet or needle to gently prick the side of your finger, producing a small drop of blood.
- Wipe away the first drop of blood with a clean tissue to ensure accuracy.

- Allow another small drop of blood to form at the puncture site.

Step 4: Applying Blood to Test Card -Carefully place a drop of blood onto each designated area on the test card, corresponding to the A, B, and Rh (D) antigens.
-Follow the instructions carefully to make sure you apply the blood correctly and can interpret the results accurately.

Step 5: Interpreting the Results
- Observe the reactions on the test card after applying the blood samples.
- A positive reaction indicates the

presence of specific antigens, determining your blood type (A, B, AB, or O) and Rh factor (positive or negative).
- Refer to the key provided with the test kit or consult with a healthcare professional to confirm your blood type.

Step 6: Understanding Your Blood Type
- Learn about the characteristics associated with your blood type, including susceptibility to certain diseases, dietary recommendations, and potential compatibility with blood transfusions.
- Explore resources such as books, articles, and reputable websites to delve deeper into the nuances of your blood type.

Step 7: Implementing Health Strategies
- Tailor your diet and lifestyle choices based on the recommendations for your blood type.
- Consider consulting with a nutritionist or healthcare provider for personalized advice and guidance.

- Incorporate exercise, stress management techniques, and other wellness practices that align with your blood type for optimal health outcomes.

Chapter 5: Understanding the Unique Characteristics of Each Blood Type

Few things are as fundamental and mysterious in the complex web of human biology as blood. Blood has a lot of information stored in its molecules, in addition to its essential functions in immune response and oxygen transport. The fact that blood may be divided into various types, each distinguished by a different combination of antigens and antibodies, is among its most fascinating features. Come along as we unravel the secrets of blood types and explore the vast array of human variations.

Body: Blood Type O
The Combatant Blood type O, also known as the "warrior" type, has its roots in the hunter-gatherer population. Type O people

have a strong immune system and a flexible metabolism, making them well-suited for survival in harsh conditions.Their ancestors thrived on a diet rich in animal proteins and plant-based foods, which still forms the cornerstone of their optimal nutrition today. Type O individuals are often described as assertive, practical, and action-oriented, embodying the warrior spirit in both body and mind.

Blood Type A
The Cultivator Blood type A has deep roots in agricultural societies, where early humans cultivated crops and formed close-knit communities. Characterized by a sensitive immune system and a tendency towards stress sensitivity, type A individuals thrive on a balanced diet rich in fruits, vegetables, and whole grains. They are known for their nurturing nature, empathy, and strong sense of social responsibility. Stress management techniques such as yoga, meditation, and

mindfulness play a crucial role in maintaining their well-being and harmony.

Blood Type B

The Nomad Blood type B represents the adventurous spirit of the nomadic tribes that roamed diverse landscapes in search of new opportunities. With a flexible immune system and a creative approach to life, type B individuals are adaptable and open-minded. They thrive on a varied diet that includes a mix of meats, dairy, grains, and vegetables. Type B personalities are characterized by their independence, curiosity, and unconventional thinking. Maintaining balance and harmony is essential for their well-being, as they navigate the ever-changing currents of life.

Blood Type AB

The Enigma Blood type AB, the rarest and most enigmatic of all, is a fusion of the characteristics of types A and B. As universal recipients, type AB individuals possess a unique blend of traits that make them adaptable and versatile. They thrive on a diet that combines elements of both vegetarian and omnivorous diets, reflecting their diverse nature. Type AB personalities are often seen as complex, creative, and empathetic, with the ability to understand and connect with people from all walks of life. Finding balance and embracing their multifaceted nature is key to their fulfillment and happiness.

Chapter 6:

What does your blood type mean for your health

There are eight blood types:
Type A-positive
Type A-negative
Type B-positive
Type B-negative
Type O-positive
Type O-negative
Type AB-positive
Type AB-negative

In the realm of human biology, blood type holds a significant role, not just for medical emergencies but also for understanding potential health risks. Let's delve into how different blood types, determined by the presence or absence of the Rh protein, can influence various aspects of health, as explained by Dr. Glenn E. Ramsey:

Heart Disease

Among the spectrum of blood types, individuals with Type O blood exhibit the lowest susceptibility to heart attacks and blood clots. This intriguing phenomenon could be attributed to higher levels of certain clotting factors in individuals with other blood types. Hence, fostering a heart-healthy lifestyle becomes paramount, especially for those with Type A, B, and AB blood.

Cancer

Research indicates a correlation between blood type and cancer risk. Individuals with Type A or Type AB blood may face a higher likelihood of developing gastric cancer, while those with Type A, B, or AB blood may have elevated risks of pancreatic cancer.

COVID-19:

Emerging studies shed light on the potential link between blood type and COVID-19 susceptibility. Preliminary findings suggest that individuals with Type A blood may be at a heightened risk of infection, whereas those with Type O blood might experience milder disease progression. Moreover, negative blood types may confer a slight advantage in terms of COVID-19 resilience. However, further research is essential to validate these observations.

Understanding one's blood type serves as a valuable tool in navigating personal health. While genetic in nature and immutable, embracing a healthy lifestyle can mitigate potential health risks associated with specific blood types. By leveraging this knowledge, individuals empower themselves to make informed decisions for optimal well-being.

Chapter 7: Personalized Nutrition: Matching Your Blood Type to Dietary Needs

Welcome to a groundbreaking approach to nutrition that goes beyond generic advice and taps into the power of your unique biology. In "Blood Type Blueprint," we delve into the revolutionary concept of personalized nutrition, where your blood type serves as a guiding light to unlock your body's full potential and achieve vibrant health like never before.

Unlock Your Body's Secrets:
Discover the fascinating link between your blood type and your body's response to different foods. From Type O to Type AB, each blood type holds valuable clues about which foods support your metabolism, enhance energy levels, and promote overall well-being.

Tailored to Thrive:
Say goodbye to one-size-fits-all diets and hello to a personalized approach that caters to your individual needs. Whether you're a Type A seeking balance, a Type B craving

variety, or a Type AB in search of harmony, we've got the tools and insights to help you thrive.

Maximize Your Energy:
Reclaim your vitality and banish fatigue with a nutrition plan designed specifically for your blood type. By fueling your body with the right foods, you can skyrocket your energy levels, boost productivity, and seize each day with renewed vigor.

Shed Excess Weight:
Bid farewell to endless dieting cycles and embrace a sustainable path to weight loss and management. With personalized nutrition, you'll discover the foods that support your body's natural metabolism, making weight loss effortless and sustainable.

Support Digestive Harmony:
Tired of digestive discomfort and bloating? Restore balance to your gut with a diet tailored to your blood type. By choosing

foods that promote digestive health, you can say goodbye to discomfort and hello to smooth, efficient digestion.

Prevent Disease, Promote Longevity:
Take control of your health destiny and reduce your risk of chronic disease with personalized nutrition. By addressing nutritional imbalances and supporting your body's natural defenses, you can safeguard your health and enjoy a life of vitality and longevity.

Part III: Implementing Blood Type Diets for Optimal Health

Chapter 8: The Blood Type A Diet: Nourishing Your Body for Balance and Vitality

Welcome to "The Blood Type A Diet: Nourishing Your Body for Balance and Vitality." In this comprehensive guide, you'll embark on a journey toward optimal health and wellness tailored specifically to your blood type. Drawing on cutting-edge research and ancient wisdom, this book offers a roadmap to transform your life through nutrition. Whether you're looking to boost energy, improve digestion, or achieve overall vitality, the Blood Type A Diet is your key to unlocking your body's full potential.

Understanding Blood Type A
Delve into the science behind blood type A and how it influences your body's needs and responses to food. Learn about the genetic and evolutionary factors that shape the Blood Type A profile and how it differs from other blood types.

The Principles of the Blood Type A Diet
Discover the foundational principles of the Blood Type A Diet, including the types of foods that support your blood type and those that should be avoided. Explore the concept of lectins and how they impact digestion and overall health for Type A individuals.

Nourishing Your Body with Type A Foods
Explore a comprehensive list of foods that are beneficial for Type A individuals, including fruits, vegetables, proteins, and grains. Learn how to create balanced meals that provide essential nutrients while aligning with your blood type.

Meal Planning and Recipes
Get practical tips for meal planning and preparation tailored to the Blood Type A Diet. Explore delicious and nutritious recipes designed to satisfy your taste buds while supporting your health goals. From breakfast to dinner and everything in between,

discover a variety of options to keep your meals exciting and fulfilling.

The Blood Type A Lifestyle

Beyond nutrition, explore holistic lifestyle practices that complement the Blood Type A Diet. From stress management techniques to exercise recommendations, discover ways to enhance your overall well-being and support your body's natural balance.

Overcoming Challenges and Staying on Track

Address common challenges faced when adopting a new dietary approach and learn strategies for staying motivated and consistent. Whether dining out, traveling, or navigating social gatherings, equip yourself with the tools to stay on track and prioritize your health.

Chapter 9:
The Blood Type B Diet: Fueling Your Body for Energy and Well-Being

The Science Behind Blood Type B and Nutrition
- Delve deeper into the scientific theories and research that underpin the Blood Type B Diet.
- Explore how blood type may influence digestion, metabolism, and overall health.
- Discuss any studies or evidence supporting the efficacy of the Blood Type B Diet.

Unveiling the Unique Dietary Needs of Blood Type B Individuals
- Identify the specific characteristics and traits associated with Blood Type B individuals.
- Explain how these traits influence dietary requirements and nutrient absorption.
- Offer insights into why certain foods may be more beneficial or detrimental for Blood Type B individuals.

Foods to Embrace: Your Ultimate Guide to Blood Type B-Friendly Choices
- Provide a comprehensive list of foods that are compatible with the Blood Type B Diet. - Highlight the nutritional benefits of these foods and how they support the health and well-being of Blood Type B individuals. - Include practical tips and recipes to help readers incorporate these foods into their diet.

Foods to Avoid: Steering Clear of Items That Don't Align with Your Blood Type
- Detail the foods that are discouraged or incompatible with the Blood Type B Diet.
- Explain the reasons behind avoiding these foods and the potential negative effects they may have on Blood Type B individuals.
- Offer alternatives or substitutions for commonly consumed foods that may not be suitable for Blood Type B individuals.

Meal Planning Made Easy: Crafting Delicious and Nutritious Blood Type B Meals

- Provide guidance on how to plan and prepare meals that adhere to the principles of the Blood Type B Diet.
- Offer tips for balancing macronutrients, incorporating a variety of foods, and creating flavorful dishes.
- Share sample meal plans and recipes to inspire and support readers in their meal planning efforts.

The Blood Type B Diet and Weight Management: Strategies for Success
- Explore the relationship between the Blood Type B Diet and weight management.
- Discuss how following this diet may support weight loss or weight maintenance goals for Blood Type B individuals.
- Offer practical strategies and tips for achieving and maintaining a healthy weight while following the Blood Type B Diet.

Enhancing Energy Levels and Vitality with the Blood Type B Diet
- Highlight the potential benefits of the Blood Type B Diet for energy levels, vitality, and overall well-being.
- Discuss how nutrient-rich foods and balanced meals can support sustained energy throughout the day.
- Provide lifestyle recommendations and practices that complement the dietary principles of the Blood Type B Diet to enhance vitality and overall health.

The Blood Type B Diet and Disease Prevention: Harnessing the Power of Nutrition for Health
- Explore the role of the Blood Type B Diet in disease prevention and health promotion.
- Discuss how dietary choices can impact risk factors for various health conditions and diseases.

- Highlight specific nutrients or food groups that may be particularly beneficial for preventing or managing certain health conditions in Blood Type B individuals.

Beyond the Plate: Incorporating Lifestyle Factors into Your Blood Type B Journey
- Acknowledge that diet is just one aspect of a healthy lifestyle and well-being.
- Discuss the importance of other lifestyle factors such as physical activity, stress management, sleep, and social connections.
- Offer practical tips and strategies for incorporating these lifestyle factors into a holistic approach to health and wellness for Blood Type B individuals.

Overcoming Challenges and Staying Committed to Your Blood Type B Lifestyle
- Address common challenges or obstacles that individuals may encounter when following the Blood Type B Diet.
- Offer strategies for overcoming these challenges and staying motivated and committed to the dietary guidelines.
- Provide encouragement and support for readers who may be navigating their Blood Type B journey and facing setbacks or difficulties.

Success Stories and Testimonials: Real-Life Experiences of Thriving on the Blood Type B Diet
- Share inspiring success stories and testimonials from individuals who have experienced positive results following the Blood Type B Diet.

- Highlight the diverse experiences and journeys of different individuals and how they have embraced and benefited from this dietary approach.
- Provide encouragement and motivation for readers by showcasing real-life examples of the transformative power of the Blood Type B Diet.

Chapter 10:
The Blood Type AB Diet: Harmonizing Your Body for Optimal Health

In this pivotal chapter, we delve deep into the transformative power of the Blood Type AB Diet, exploring how it harmonizes your body to unlock the gateway to optimal health. The Blood Type AB Diet is not just a dietary plan; it's a holistic approach to nourishing your body, mind, and spirit, tailored specifically to your unique blood type.

Understanding Your Blood Type AB:
Blood Type AB individuals are often described as the "universal recipients" due to their adaptable nature. This adaptability extends beyond their blood type to their dietary requirements. Understanding your Blood Type AB means recognizing the nuances of your body's needs, embracing your innate adaptability, and harnessing it to achieve optimal health and vitality.

The Science Behind the Blood Type AB Diet:

The foundation of the Blood Type AB Diet lies in the groundbreaking research of Dr. Peter J. D'Adamo and the emerging field of nutrigenomics. This science explores how our genes interact with the foods we eat, influencing everything from digestion to disease risk. By understanding the intricate relationship between your blood type and nutrition, you can unlock the secrets to optimal health and well-being.

Principles of the Blood Type AB Diet:

At the core of the Blood Type AB Diet are principles designed to harmonize your body and support its natural balance. These principles emphasize the consumption of whole, nutrient-rich foods while avoiding those that may disrupt your body's harmony. By following these guidelines, you can nourish your body from the inside out, promoting vitality and longevity.

Embracing Blood Type AB-Friendly Foods:
Discover the vibrant array of foods that are compatible with the Blood Type AB Diet. From nutrient-dense fruits and vegetables to lean proteins and healthy fats, these foods provide the essential nutrients your body needs to thrive. By embracing these foods, you can fuel your body with the building blocks of health and vitality.

Steering Clear of Disruptive Foods:
Navigate the pitfalls of the modern diet by identifying and avoiding foods that may disrupt your body's harmony. Processed foods, refined sugars, and inflammatory ingredients can wreak havoc on your health, leading to digestive issues, inflammation, and chronic disease. By steering clear of these disruptive foods, you can support your body's natural balance and well-being.

Crafting Blood Type AB Meals:
Empower yourself in the kitchen by learning how to craft delicious and nutritious meals that align with the Blood Type AB Diet. From simple meal prep techniques to flavorful recipe ideas, discover how to create meals that nourish your body and satisfy your taste buds. By embracing a variety of foods and flavors, you can enjoy a diverse and satisfying diet that supports your health and vitality.

Achieving Weight Management and Vitality:
Unlock the secrets to achieving and maintaining a healthy weight on the Blood Type AB Diet. By nourishing your body with nutrient-rich foods and embracing a balanced approach to eating, you can support your metabolism, manage your weight, and enhance your energy levels. With vitality as your guide, you can thrive in every aspect of your life.

Embracing Holistic Wellness:
Embrace a holistic approach to wellness by nurturing your body, mind, and spirit. From stress management techniques to mindfulness practices, discover how to cultivate balance and harmony in every aspect of your life. By integrating lifestyle factors into your Blood Type AB journey, you can enhance your well-being and live your best life.

Chapter 11:
Strengthening Your Body for Longevity and Wellness

Unlock the Secrets to Longevity and Wellness with the Blood Type O Diet. In this pivotal chapter, we delve into the transformative power of nutrition tailored specifically to Blood Type O individuals. Discover how to strengthen your body, enhance your vitality, and unlock the keys to a lifetime of optimal health and well-being.

Introduction to the Blood Type O Diet:
Welcome to the gateway to longevity and wellness. The Blood Type O Diet is not just a dietary plan; it's a lifestyle approach designed to support your body's unique needs and unlock your full potential. In this chapter, we'll explore the principles and

strategies that will empower you to thrive on the Blood Type O Diet and live your best life.

Understanding Blood Type O:
Blood Type O individuals are often described as the "original blood type," with ancestral roots dating back to hunter-gatherer societies. As such, they thrive on a diet rich in animal proteins, vegetables, and fruits, with limited grains and dairy. Understanding the evolutionary context of your blood type is key to optimizing your health and well-being.

The Science Behind the Blood Type O Diet:
Delve into the science behind the Blood Type O Diet and uncover the research supporting its efficacy. From the pioneering work of Dr. Peter J. D'Adamo to the latest studies in nutrigenomics, explore how your blood type influences everything from digestion to disease risk. By understanding the science, you can harness the power of nutrition to support your long-term health goals.

Principles of the Blood Type O Diet:
At the heart of the Blood Type O Diet are principles designed to strengthen your body and promote longevity. These principles emphasize the consumption of lean proteins, fruits, and vegetables, while minimizing grains, legumes, and dairy. By aligning your diet with these principles, you can optimize your health and vitality for years to come.

Embracing Blood Type O-Friendly Foods:
Discover the diverse array of foods that are compatible with the Blood Type O Diet. From lean meats and fish to leafy greens and berries, these foods provide the essential nutrients your body needs to thrive. By embracing these foods, you can fuel your body with the building blocks of health and support your longevity goals.

Avoiding Disruptive Foods:
Navigate the modern food landscape by identifying and avoiding foods that may disrupt your body's natural balance. Processed foods, refined sugars, and certain grains can lead to inflammation, digestive issues, and chronic disease in Blood Type O individuals. By steering clear of these disruptive foods, you can support your body's natural resilience and well-being.

Crafting Blood Type O Meals:
Empower yourself in the kitchen by learning how to craft delicious and nutritious meals that align with the Blood Type O Diet. From hearty salads to savory stir-fries, discover how to create meals that nourish your body and delight your taste buds. By embracing a variety of flavors and textures, you can enjoy a diverse and satisfying diet that supports your longevity and wellness goals.

Achieving Longevity and Wellness:
Unlock the secrets to longevity and wellness on the Blood Type O Diet. By nourishing your body with nutrient-rich foods and adopting a balanced approach to eating, you can support your metabolism, maintain a healthy weight, and enhance your energy levels. With vitality as your guide, you can thrive in every aspect of your life and embrace the gift of longevity.

Embracing Holistic Wellness:
Embrace a holistic approach to wellness by nurturing your body, mind, and spirit. From regular exercise to stress management techniques, discover journeys, you can enhance your well-being and cultivate a sense of vitality and purpose.

Part IV: Practical Strategies and Meal Plans

Chapter 12:

Shopping Smart.

How to cultivate balance and harmony in every aspect of your life. By integrating lifestyle factors into your Blood Type O : Grocery Tips for Your Blood Type:

In this chapter, we delve into the intriguing world of personalized nutrition by aligning our grocery choices with our blood type. This innovative approach to shopping not only promises a healthier lifestyle but also opens up a realm of possibilities for optimizing our well-being.

Imagine walking through the aisles of your local grocery store with newfound clarity, armed with the knowledge of which foods harmonize best with your unique blood type. For Type A individuals, leaning towards a plant-based diet rich in fruits, vegetables, and whole grains can be transformative. The vibrant colors of fresh produce beckon, promising vitality and energy tailored to your genetic makeup.

Type B personalities, on the other hand, might find solace in a more varied diet that includes a balance of lean meats, dairy, and an array of fruits and vegetables. Embracing the versatility of their blood type, they navigate the aisles with confidence, selecting ingredients that not only nourish their bodies but also tantalize their taste buds.

For those with Type AB blood, the grocery store becomes a playground of culinary experimentation. With a blend of traits from Types A and B, individuals of this blood type can explore a diverse range of foods, from tofu to seafood, unlocking a world of gastronomic delights tailored to their unique physiology.

And let's not forget about the stalwart Type O individuals, whose ancestral roots call for a hearty diet reminiscent of hunter-gatherer days. Laden with lean meats, fish, and robust greens, their shopping carts are a testament to strength and vitality, reflecting their evolutionary heritage with every selection.

But shopping smart goes beyond mere adherence to blood type guidelines; it's about making informed choices that nourish both body and soul. It's about selecting organic, locally sourced produce whenever possible, supporting sustainability and environmental stewardship. It's about prioritizing whole, unprocessed foods over their overly refined counterparts, reclaiming our connection to the earth and its bounty.

In a world inundated with fad diets and conflicting nutritional advice, the concept of shopping smart based on blood type offers a refreshing perspective rooted in science and personalized wellness. It empowers individuals to take control of their health journey, one grocery trip at a time, forging a path towards vitality, longevity, and fulfillment.

CHAPTER 13:
Right Recipes Different Blood Type

Here, we embark on a culinary journey that celebrates the diversity of our blood types through the lens of delicious and nutritious recipes. From tantalizing appetizers to mouthwatering mains and decadent desserts, these dishes are carefully crafted to cater to the unique nutritional needs of each blood type, promising a symphony of flavors and a bounty of health benefits.

For Type A individuals, we present a tantalizing array of plant-based recipes that embrace the bounty of nature's harvest. From vibrant salads bursting with color and nutrients to hearty grain bowls infused with aromatic herbs and spices, these dishes nourish the body and soul, reflecting the ethos of balance and harmony that defines the Type A blood type.

Type B personalities will delight in the eclectic mix of recipes that cater to their versatile palate. From succulent stir-fries teeming with fresh vegetables and lean proteins to savory stews brimming with hearty grains and legumes, these dishes offer a feast for the senses, celebrating the adventurous spirit and adaptable nature of the Type B blood type.

For those with Type AB blood, we present a fusion of flavors that marries the best of both worlds. From innovative sushi rolls that combine seafood with crisp vegetables to inventive salads that blend sweet and savory elements, these recipes embody the spirit of creativity and experimentation that defines the Type AB blood type.

And let's not forget about the stalwart Type O individuals, whose ancestral roots inspire a menu of robust and satisfying fare. From sizzling steaks seasoned to perfection to zesty salads adorned with tangy dressings, these dishes honor the primal instincts and robust constitution of the Type O blood type, offering sustenance and satisfaction in equal measure.

But beyond mere culinary indulgence, these recipes are designed with health and wellness in mind. Each dish is thoughtfully curated to optimize digestion, support immune function, and promote overall vitality, harnessing the power of food as medicine to nourish and heal from the inside out.

In a world awash with dietary dogma and one-size-fits-all approaches to nutrition, the concept of Right Recipes Different Blood Type offers a refreshing perspective rooted in individuality and customization. It empowers individuals to embrace their genetic heritage and celebrate the unique characteristics that make them who they are, one delectable dish at a time.

Blood Type and Suitable Recipes

Type O
Lean meats like beef, lamb, and poultry. Vegetables like spinach, broccoli, and kale. Fruits like berries, plums, and figs.

Type A
Plant-based proteins like tofu and tempeh. Vegetables like spinach, broccoli, and carrots. Fruits like berries, apples, and grapes.

Type B
Lean meats like lamb and turkey. Dairy like yogurt and cheese. Vegetables like cabbage, carrots, and sweet potatoes. Fruits like bananas, grapes, and pineapple.

Type AB
Seafood like salmon and mackerel. Dairy like yogurt and cheese. Vegetables like spinach, kale, and broccoli. Fruits like berries, plums, and pineapple.

Part V: Enhancing Your Lifestyle with Blood Type Diets

Chapter 14:
Fitness and Exercise: Tailoring Workouts to Your Blood Type

In Chapter 14, we embark on an exhilarating exploration of fitness and exercise, guided by the principle of tailoring workouts to match our unique blood types. Gone are the days of generic exercise routines that leave us feeling uninspired and unfulfilled. Instead, we embrace a holistic approach to physical activity that honors our genetic predispositions and maximizes our potential for health and vitality.

ForTypeAindividuals,weadvocateforgentle,mindfulformsof exercise that promote flexibility, balance, and inner peace. From the graceful movements of yoga to the flowing sequences of tai chi, these disciplines not only strengthen the body but also calm the mind, aligning perfectly with the serene nature of the Type A blood type.

Type B personalities, with their adventurous spirit and boundless energy, thrive on dynamic, varied workouts that keep them engaged and motivated. From high-intensity interval training to outdoor activities like hiking and cycling, these individuals revel in the challenge of pushing their limits and exploring new horizons, reflecting the bold and adventurous nature of the Type B blood type.

For those with Type AB blood, we advocate for a balanced approach to fitness that combines elements of both strength training and mind-body practices. From Pilates sessions that sculpt and tone the body to dance classes that ignite the spirit and invigorate the soul, these workouts celebrate the duality of the Type AB blood type, promoting harmony and balance in both body and mind.

And let's not forget about the indomitable Type O individuals, whose primal instincts and robust constitution call for intense, high-impact workouts that channel their inner warrior. From weightlifting sessions that build strength and power to martial arts practices that cultivate discipline and focus, these individuals thrive on the challenge of pushing their bodies to the limit, reflecting the tenacious and resilient nature of the Type O blood type.

But beyond mere physical exertion, these tailored workouts are designed to optimize health and well-being on a deeper level. Each exercise regimen is carefully curated to support immune function, improve cardiovascular health, and enhance overall vitality, harnessing the power of movement to promote longevity and resilience from the inside out.

In a world obsessed with one-size-fits-all fitness trends and fleeting fads, the concept of Tailoring Workouts to Your Blood Type offers a refreshing alternative rooted in science and personalized wellness. It empowers individuals to embrace their genetic heritage and celebrate the unique characteristics that make them who they are, one workout at a time.

Chapter 15:
Stress Management: Holistic Approaches for Each Blood Type

We look into the art of stress management, offering a comprehensive guide to holistic approaches tailored to the unique needs of each blood type. In today's fast-paced world, where stress has become an inevitable part of daily life, it's more important than ever to equip ourselves with effective strategies for mitigating its impact and promoting inner peace and well-being.

ForTypeAindividuals,whoareoftenpronetooverthinkingand internalizing stress, we advocate for practices that promote relaxation and mindfulness. From meditation and deep breathing exercises to gentle yoga and tai chi, these techniques help quiet the mind, soothe the nervous system, and cultivate a sense of inner calm, aligning perfectly with the serene nature of the Type A blood type.

Type B personalities, with their adventurous spirit and spontaneous nature, thrive on activities that engage both mind and body in equal measure. From outdoor pursuits like hiking and gardening to creative endeavors like painting and music, these individuals find solace in activities that allow them to express themselves freely and connect with the world around them, reflecting the dynamic and adaptable nature of the Type B blood type.

For those with Type AB blood, we advocate for a balanced approach to stress management that integrates elements of both introspection and engagement. From journaling and visualization exercises to volunteer work and social activities, these individuals benefit from a holistic approach that addresses the multifaceted nature of stress, promoting harmony and equilibrium in both mind and spirit.

And let's not forget about the resilient Type O individuals, whose strong and determined nature enables them to confront stress head-on with courage and fortitude. From vigorous exercise sessions that release tension and boost endorphins to practical problem-solving techniques that empower them to take control of their circumstances, these individuals thrive in the face of adversity, reflecting the tenacious and resilient nature of the Type O blood type.

But beyond mere coping mechanisms, these holistic approaches to stress management are designed to promote overall well-being and vitality on a deeper level. By addressing the root causes of stress and fostering a sense of balance and harmony within, they empower individuals to navigate life's challenges with grace and resilience, unlocking the full potential of health and happiness.

In a world where stress has become an epidemic, the concept of Holistic Approaches for Each Blood Type offers a beacon of hope and empowerment. It reminds us that we are not powerless victims of our circumstances but active agents in our own healing and transformation, capable of cultivating inner peace and well-being regardless of the challenges we face.

Chapter 16:
Integrating Mental Health with Blood Type Nutrition

We embark on a groundbreaking exploration of the intersection between mental health and nutrition, weaving together the latest research findings with the principles of blood type nutrition to offer a holistic approach to emotional well-being. In a world where stress, anxiety, and depression have reached epidemic proportions, it's more important than ever to recognize the profound impact that diet and lifestyle choices can have on our mental health.

For Type A individuals, who are often sensitive and introspective by nature, we advocate for a diet rich in plant-based foods and mindfulness practices that promote serenity and balance. From nourishing soups and salads to soothing herbal teas and meditation exercises, these techniques help calm the mind, soothe the soul, and alleviate the symptoms of anxiety and stress, aligning perfectly with the tranquil nature of the Type A blood type.

Type B personalities, with their dynamic and adventurous spirit, benefit from a balanced diet that includes a variety of foods and activities that stimulate both body and mind. From hearty stir-fries and colorful smoothie bowls to outdoor adventures and creative pursuits, these individuals thrive on a diverse range of experiences that engage their senses and ignite their passion for life, reflecting the vibrant and adaptable nature of the Type B blood type.

For those with Type AB blood, we advocate for a holistic approach to mental health that integrates elements of both introspection and engagement. From journaling and visualization exercises to volunteer work and social activities, these individuals benefit from a multifaceted approach that addresses the complex interplay between mind, body, and spirit, promoting harmony and balance on all levels.

And let's not forget about the resilient Type O individuals, whose strong and determined nature enables them to confront mental health challenges with courage and fortitude. From vigorous exercise sessions that release tension and boost endorphins to practical problem-solving techniques that empower them to take control of their thoughts and emotions, these individuals thrive in the face of adversity, reflecting the tenacious and resilient nature of the Type O blood type.

But beyond mere symptom management, the integration of mental health with blood type nutrition offers a path to true healing and transformation. By addressing the underlying imbalances and deficiencies that contribute to mental health issues, we empower individuals to reclaim their sense of well-being and vitality, unlocking the full potential of a life lived in harmony with their genetic blueprint.

In a world where mental health is too often overlooked or stigmatized, the concept of Integrating Mental Health with Blood Type Nutrition offers a beacon of hope and empowerment. It reminds us that we are not defined by our diagnoses or limitations but by our capacity for resilience, growth, and self-discovery.

PartVI: Enhancing Your Health Plans

Chapter 17:
Supplements and Support

In the realm of blood type diets, understanding the nuances of your blood type's nutritional requirements is paramount. While adhering to a diet tailored to your blood type forms the foundation of your wellness journey, supplementing with targeted nutrients and embracing comprehensive support systems can amplify the benefits and propel you towards optimal health.

Filling Nutritional Gaps: Blood Type Specific Supplementation

Each blood type possesses unique dietary needs and tolerances, and supplements can play a crucial role in addressing these individualized requirements. For instance, individuals with Type O blood may benefit from supplements that support their robust metabolism and digestive health, while those with Type A blood might prioritize supplements that bolster immune function and promote stress management. By aligning supplementation with your blood type's nutritional profile, you enhance the efficacy of your dietary choices and maximize your overall well-being.

Personalized Wellness Solutions: Tailoring Supplements to Your Blood Type

Just as blood type diets emphasize personalized nutrition, so too should supplementation be tailored to suit your specific blood type. Whether you're an advocate of the blood type diet for Type A, Type B, Type AB, or Type O, integrating blood type-specific supplements can complement your dietary approach and address any potential nutritional deficiencies or imbalances. By customizing your supplement regimen to align with your blood type's unique requirements, you optimize nutrient absorption and support your body's innate ability to thrive.

Quality Matters: Selecting Supplements with Care

When incorporating supplements into your blood type diet, prioritizing quality is paramount. Look for supplements from reputable brands that adhere to rigorous quality control standards and third-party testing protocols. Additionally, seek guidance from healthcare professionals or certified nutritionists who can provide personalized recommendations based on your blood type and health goals. By investing in high-quality supplements that are tailored to your blood type's specific needs, you ensure that you're receiving the most effective support for your wellness journey.

Holistic Support Systems: Integrating Supplements with Lifestyle Practices

While supplements are a valuable component of a blood type diet, they are most effective when integrated into a holistic support system that addresses all aspects of well-being. Incorporating lifestyle practices such as regular exercise, stress management techniques, adequate sleep, and mindful eating habits synergizes with supplementation to optimize health outcomes. By embracing a comprehensive approach that encompasses both dietary and lifestyle factors, you empower yourself to fully harness the benefits of your blood type diet and supplements alike.

Investing in Long-Term Health: The Lucrative Returns of Blood Type-Specific Support

By prioritizing blood type-specific supplementation and embracing a holistic approach to health, you make a lucrative investment in your long-term well-being. The synergistic combination of personalized nutrition, targeted supplementation, and supportive lifestyle practices lays the foundation for vibrant health, enhanced vitality, and resilience in the face of life's challenges. As you nourish your body according to its unique blood type requirements and provide it with the support it needs to thrive, you unlock the full potential of your blood type diet and pave the way for a future characterized by optimal health and vitality.

Chapter 18:
Embracing Your Health Journey:
Motivation and Inspiration from Others

Embarking on a journey towards healthier living is a deeply personal endeavor, yet it's often the shared experiences, successes, and stories of others that provide the spark of inspiration needed to ignite our own transformation. In the realm of blood type diets for healthy living, drawing motivation from the journeys of fellow individuals navigating similar paths can be a powerful catalyst for success. Let us delve into the stories of those who have embraced their health journeys, finding motivation, inspiration, and invaluable insights along the way.

Discovering Shared Experiences: Connecting Through Stories

As you embark on your blood type diet journey, you're not alone. Countless individuals around the world are also exploring the transformative power of aligning their dietary choices with their blood type. By immersing yourself in the stories of others who have walked similar paths, you gain a sense of camaraderie and solidarity that fuels your own determination.

Whether it's through online communities, support groups, or personal testimonials, hearing how others have overcome challenges, achieved milestones, and experienced tangible improvements in their health can instill a sense of hope and possibility in your own journey.

Finding Role Models: Inspiring Examples of Success

Within the realm of blood type diets, there exist inspiring individuals who have not only embraced the principles of personalized nutrition but have also thrived as a result. From celebrities to everyday individuals, these role models serve as beacons of inspiration, demonstrating the transformative potential of aligning diet with blood type. Whether it's witnessing a public figure share their journey to better health or hearing the remarkable stories of ordinary people achieving extraordinary results, these examples of success fuel your motivation and remind you of the profound impact that lifestyle choices can have on overall well-being.

Sharing Successes and Challenges: Building a Supportive Community

In the pursuit of optimal health through the blood type diet, sharing successes, challenges, and insights with others fosters a sense of community and mutual support. Whether it's celebrating a milestone, seeking advice during a plateau, or offering words of encouragement to fellow travelers on the journey, the connections forged within a supportive community provide invaluable motivation and accountability. By surrounding yourself with like-minded individuals who share your commitment to health and wellness, you create a network of support that propels you forward and reinforces your dedication to living your best life.

Inspiring Transformational Tales: Stories of Resilience and Renewal

Within every health journey lies a narrative of resilience, determination, and transformation. From overcoming health obstacles to reclaiming vitality and vitality, the stories of individuals on the blood type diet are rich with inspiration and insight. Whether it's witnessing someone reverse chronic health conditions, achieve weight loss goals, or simply experience a newfound sense of energy and well-being, these tales of transformation serve as reminders of the incredible potential that lies within each of us. By embracing these stories with an open heart and a receptive mind, you glean valuable lessons, strategies, and encouragement to fuel your own journey towards optimal health.

Harnessing the Power of Shared Experience: Your Journey, Your Inspiration

As you embark on your own health journey through the blood type diet, remember that you are part of a vibrant and supportive community united by a shared commitment to well-being. Draw inspiration from the stories of others, celebrate your successes, and find strength in moments of challenge. Your journey is unique, yet it is enriched by the collective wisdom and encouragement of those who have walked similar paths. Embrace the power of shared experience, and let the stories of others ignite the flame of motivation within you as you continue to pursue a life of vibrant health and vitality through the blood type diet.

Part VII: Troubleshooting and FAQs**

Chapter 19:
Common Challenges and Solutions on Blood Type Diets

We confront the common challenges faced by individuals embarking on a blood type diet journey and offer innovative solutions to overcome them. While the promise of improved health and vitality through personalized nutrition is enticing, navigating the complexities and nuances of implementing a blood type diet can sometimes be daunting. That's why we've compiled a comprehensive guide to help you navigate the pitfalls and pitfalls and pave the way for success.

One of the most common challenges faced by individuals on a blood type diet is the difficulty of finding suitable foods that align with their specific blood type recommendations. With so many conflicting dietary guidelines and food options available, it can be overwhelming to know where to start. That's why we've curated an extensive list of blood type-friendly foods and meal ideas to inspire and empower you on your journey. From vibrant salads and hearty stews to decadent desserts and satisfying snacks, there's something for everyone, regardless of blood type.

Another challenge that individuals may encounter is the temptation to stray from their blood type diet plan, especially in social situations or when dining out. It can be challenging to resist the allure of forbidden foods or to navigate unfamiliar menus without compromising your dietary principles. That's why we've developed a range of practical strategies and tips to help you stay on track and make informed choices in any situation. From pre-planning meals and snacks to communicating your dietary needs with confidence, we've got you covered every step of the way.

Furthermore, some individuals may struggle with the transition to a blood type diet, experiencing detox symptoms or temporary discomfort as their body adjusts to new dietary patterns. While these challenges can be disheartening, they are often a sign that your body is responding positively to the changes you're making. To help you navigate this transition period with ease, we've compiled a list of supportive practices and remedies to help alleviate symptoms and promote overall well-being. From gentle detoxifying teas to soothing self-care rituals, we're here to support you on your journey to optimal health.

And let's not forget about the emotional challenges that can arise when embarking on a blood type diet journey. It's natural to feel overwhelmed or frustrated at times, especially when faced with setbacks or obstacles along the way. That's why we've included a range of empowering resources and tools to help you cultivate resilience, motivation, and self-compassion as you navigate the ups and downs of your health journey.

From inspirational affirmations and guided meditations to supportive online communities and expert advice, we're here to cheer you on every step of the way.

In a world filled with dietary confusion and misinformation, the concept of Common Challenges and Solutions on Blood Type Diets offers a beacon of hope and empowerment. It reminds us that while the path to optimal health may not always be easy, it is always worth pursuing. With the right knowledge, support, and mindset, you can overcome any obstacle and thrive on your blood type diet journey.

Chapter 20:
Frequently Asked Questions About Blood Type Nutrition

This serves as your ultimate guide to navigating the world of blood type nutrition by addressing the most frequently asked questions and concerns. As you embark on your journey towards optimal health and vitality, it's natural to have questions about the principles, practices, and potential benefits of aligning your diet with your blood type. That's why we've compiled this comprehensive FAQ to provide clarity, insight, and guidance every step of the way.

Question 1: What is blood type nutrition, and how does it work?
Answer: Blood type nutrition is a dietary approach that tailors food choices and eating habits to match an individual's blood

type. Proponents believe that each blood type (A, B, AB, O) has unique nutritional needs and tolerances based on ancestral and

genetic factors. By following a diet specific to their blood type, individuals can optimize digestion, support immune function, and promote overall health and well-being.

Question 2: How do I determine my blood type?
Answer: Your blood type can be determined through a simple blood test performed by a healthcare professional. Alternatively, there are at-home blood typing kits available for purchase that allow you to determine your blood type using a small sample of blood.

Question 3: What foods are recommended for each blood type?

Answer: The recommended foods for each blood type vary based on individual characteristics and genetic predispositions. However, some general guidelines include:

- Type A: Emphasize plant-based foods such as fruits, vegetables, and whole grains.

- Type B: Include a balance of lean meats, dairy, fruits, and vegetables.

- Type AB: Enjoy a varied diet that includes a mix of foods from both Type A and Type B recommendations.

- Type O: Focus on lean meats, fish, fruits, and vegetables, with limited grains and dairy.

Question 4: Are there specific foods I should avoid based on my blood type?

Answer: Yes, proponents of blood type nutrition suggest avoiding certain foods that may be less compatible with your blood type. For example, Type A individuals may be advised to limit animal products and processed foods, while Type O individuals may benefit from avoiding dairy and gluten-containing grains.

Question 5: Is there scientific evidence to support blood type nutrition?

Answer: While the concept of blood type nutrition is based on scientific principles, research supporting its efficacy is still evolving. Some studies have shown associations between blood type and certain health outcomes, but more research is needed to fully understand the implications of blood type on dietary needs and responses.

Question 6: Can blood type nutrition help with weight loss?
Answer: Some individuals may experience weight loss or improved body composition when following a blood type-specific diet, particularly if it aligns with their individual needs and preferences. However, weight loss results can vary depending on factors such as overall diet quality, lifestyle habits, and genetic predispositions.

Question 7: Can I still follow a blood type diet if I have dietary restrictions or food allergies?

Answer: Yes, blood type nutrition can be adapted to accommodate dietary restrictions or food allergies. By focusing on foods that are compatible with your blood type and substituting alternatives for problematic foods, you can still reap the benefits of a personalized diet while meeting your individual dietary needs.

Question 8: Are there any potential risks or drawbacks to following a blood type diet?

Answer: While many people find success and improved health outcomes with blood type nutrition, it's essential to approach any dietary change with caution and awareness. Some individuals may experience challenges such as nutrient deficiencies, social limitations, or difficulty adhering to restrictive dietary guidelines. Consulting with a healthcare professional or registered dietitian can help mitigate risks and ensure a balanced and sustainable approach to blood type nutrition.

Conclusion

The journey through the pages of "Blood Type Diets" unveils a transformative path towards a healthier future, illuminated by the guiding principles of personalized nutrition. From the foundational concepts of aligning dietary choices with blood type to the practical strategies for navigating common challenges and questions, this book serves as a beacon of hope and empowerment for those seeking to optimize their health and vitality.

As we've explored the unique dietary recommendations tailored to each blood type, we've discovered a profound connection between our genetic blueprint and the foods that nourish our bodies and minds. Whether you're a Type A seeking serenity through plant-based fare, a Type B embracing adventure and variety, a Type AB balancing duality and creativity, or a Type O channeling primal strength and resilience, the principles of blood type nutrition offer a personalized roadmap to wellness that honors our individuality and empowers us to thrive.

Through chapters dedicated to shopping smart, right recipes, fitness and exercise, stress management, mental health integration, and addressing common challenges, we've uncovered a holistic approach to health and well-being that transcends the limitations of one-size-fits-all dietary advice. By embracing the wisdom of blood type nutrition, we unlock the door to a healthier future filled with vitality, resilience, and joy.

Imagine a world where every trip to the grocery store is an opportunity to nourish your body and soul according to your unique genetic blueprint. Picture a life where every meal is a celebration of vibrant flavors and nourishing ingredients that support your health and well-being. Envision a future where stress is managed with grace and resilience, and mental health is nurtured through mindful practices and self-care rituals tailored to your individual needs.

This is the promise of "Blood Type Diets": a future where optimal health and vitality are within reach for all who dare to embrace the transformative power of personalized nutrition. As we bid farewell to the pages of this book, let us carry forth the lessons learned and the wisdom gained on our journey towards a healthier, happier, and more vibrant life. For in the embrace of blood type nutrition lies the key to unlocking our full potential and realizing our dreams of a brighter tomorrow. Let us step boldly into this future, guided by the knowledge that our genetic blueprint holds the key to our health and vitality. After all, when it comes to our well-being, the future is ours to shape, and the possibilities are limitless.

Appendix

Congratulations on taking the first steps towards achieving optimal health and vitality through blood type nutrition! To further support you on your journey, we've curated a list of additional resources and references that will help deepen your understanding and broaden your knowledge.

1. Books

Eat Right for Your Type* by Dr. Peter J. D'Adamo:
This groundbreaking book introduced the concept of blood type nutrition, offering comprehensive guidance on tailoring your diet to your specific blood type.

Cook Right for Your Type by Dr. Peter J. D'Adamo:
A companion cookbook filled with mouthwatering recipes and meal plans designed for each blood type, making it easier to incorporate blood type nutrition into your daily life.

Live Right for Your Type by Dr. Peter J. D'Adamo:
An insightful exploration of how blood type influences not only dietary needs but also exercise, stress management, and overall lifestyle choices.

2. Websites and Online Communities

Blood Type Diet Official Website
(www.dadamo.com): A valuable resource offering information, articles, and updates on blood type nutrition, authored by Dr. Peter J. D'Adamo himself.

Blood Type Diet Forums:
Connect with fellow enthusiasts, share experiences, and find support on your blood type diet journey through online forums and social media groups dedicated to blood type nutrition.

3. Nutritional Supplements

- **Blood Type Specific Supplements**: Explore a range of supplements formulated for each blood type to address potential deficiencies and support overall health and well-being.

4. Healthcare Professionals

Naturopathic Doctors:
Consult with a naturopathic doctor specializing in blood type nutrition and personalized wellness for tailored guidance and support.

Registered Dietitians:
Work with a registered dietitian knowledgeable about blood type nutrition to develop a customized meal plan aligned with your blood type recommendations.

5. Research Studies and Scientific Articles

PubMed (www.ncbi.nlm.nih.gov/pubmed): Search for research studies and articles on blood type nutrition, dietary interventions, and health outcomes to stay informed about the latest advancements.

6. Cookbooks and Recipe Websites

Blood Type Diet Recipe Books:
Explore a variety of cookbooks and recipe websites offering delicious and nutritious meals tailored to your blood type.

By utilizing these additional resources and references, you can deepen your understanding of blood type nutrition, access valuable support, and enhance your journey towards optimal health and vitality. Remember, knowledge is power, and with the right tools and resources, you can unlock the full potential of personalized nutrition for a healthier, happier life.

Happy reading and bon appétit!